FROM STRUGGLING TO FINDING STRENGTH:

A Survivor's Guide to Life After

Breast Cancer

Janet martins

Contents

DISCLAIMER:

All content is provided as general information only, and should not be taken as medical advice or professional guidance. Please consult with a qualified healthcare provider if you have any questions or concerns about your individual situation.

INTRODUCTION

When you are first diagnosed with breast cancer, it feels like your world is crashing down around you. All of a sudden, you have to worry about treatments, surgeries, and the possibility of losing your hair or your breasts. It is a lot to take in. But eventually, you come to terms with the diagnosis and start fighting for your life. This is just the beginning of your journey. There will be good days and bad days, but eventually, you learn to live again. In this book, we will discuss what life is like after breast cancer. We will talk about the struggles that survivors face and how they find strength in the face of adversity.

If you are a breast cancer survivor, then you know that the journey is far from over when you finish treatment. There are many challenges that come along with life after cancer, but there is also great strength to be found in overcoming them.

In this book, we will discuss some of the things that survivors can do to find their new normal and live a fulfilling life after cancer. We hope that this information will help give you the strength to face whatever comes your way!

PART ONE

WHAT IS BREAST CANCER?

With the disorder known as breast cancer, the cells in the breast begin to develop in an uncontrolled manner. There are several subtypes of breast cancer to be aware of. The kind of breast cancer that a woman has is determined by which cells in her breast become cancer.

Cancer of the breast may originate in a variety of locations inside the breast. There are three primary components that make up a breast: the lobules, the ducts, and the connective tissue. The lobules contain the glands that are responsible for milk production. The milk is transported to the nipple through tubes known as ducts. Everything is surrounded by connective tissue, which is made up of both fibrous and fatty tissue, and it is what keeps everything together. The majority of breast cancers start in the ducts or lobules of the breast.

Blood arteries and lymph vessels are two potential pathways by which breast cancer might move outside the breast. Metastasis is the term used to describe the process by which breast cancer spreads to different areas of the body.

Cancer of the breast is a disease that begins in the breast and is most often caused by a malignant tumor. A clump of cells that develops in an uncontrolled manner is referred to be a malignant tumor. It is also possible for the malignant cells to metastasis, which means to spread to other tissues or areas of the body.

There are three distinct forms of breast tissue: lobules, ducts, and connective tissue. Any one of them may become infected with cancer.

The vast majority of cancers start in either the lobules, which are the milk-producing glands, or the ducts, which are the passageways down which milk goes to the nipple. Nevertheless, tumors may also grow in the fibrous and fatty connective tissue that surrounds the lobules and ducts. This is another possible location for tumor development.

SIGNS AND SYMPTOMS

Breast cancer most commonly presents as a painless lump or thickening in the breast. It is important that women finding an abnormal lump in the breast consult a health practitioner without a delay of more than 1-2 months even when there is no pain associated with it. Seeking medical attention at the first sign of a potential symptom allows for more successful treatment.

Generally, symptoms of breast cancer include:

- a breast lump or thickening;

- alteration in size, shape, or appearance of a breast;
- dimpling, redness, pitting, or other alteration in the skin;
- change in nipple appearance or alteration in the skin surrounding the nipple (areola); and/or
- abnormal nipple discharge.

The development of lumps in the breast may occur for a variety of causes, the most majority of which are not related to cancer. Up to ninety percent of breast tumors do not have malignant cells. Breast infections and benign lumps like fibroadenomas and cysts fall within the category of breast abnormalities that are not malignant.

Since breast cancer may manifest in such a broad range of different ways, it is essential to get a comprehensive medical evaluation. Tests, such as imaging of the breast and, in certain situations, tissue collection (biopsy), should be performed on women who have persistent abnormalities (usually lasting more than one month) to identify whether a lump is malignant (cancerous) or benign.

Although while advanced malignancies may erode through the skin and generate open sores (also known as an ulcer), the condition is not always excruciatingly painful. A breast biopsy is something that should be done for women who have breast sores that do not heal.

Breast cancers have the potential to metastasize, or spread, to other parts of the body, as well as cause additional symptoms. While it is possible to have cancer-bearing lymph nodes that cannot be touched, the lymph nodes located under the arm are often the first identifiable site of dissemination when the disease has moved elsewhere in the body.

Cancerous cells have the potential to spread to other organs over the course of time, including the lungs, liver, brain, and bones. New cancer-related symptoms, such as pain in the bones or headaches, may manifest themselves as the cancer cells reach these places.

WHO IS AT RISK?

There is no evidence that breast cancer may be passed on to others or that it is an infectious illness. In contrast to other cancers that are known to have infectious origins, such as human papillomavirus (HPV) infection and cervical cancer, there are no known infectious factors that contribute to the development of breast cancer. This is true of both viral and bacterial infections.

It is estimated that almost half of all breast cancers occur in women who have no other recognized breast cancer risk factors than being female and becoming older (over 40 years). Age, obesity, harmful use of alcohol, a family history of breast cancer, a history of radiation exposure, reproductive history (such as age that menstrual periods began and age at first pregnancy), tobacco use, and postmenopausal hormone therapy are all factors that can increase the risk of developing breast cancer.

Behavioral choices and related interventions that reduce the risk of breast cancer include:

- prolonged breastfeeding;
- regular physical activity;
- weight control;
- avoidance of harmful use of alcohol;
- avoidance of exposure to tobacco smoke;
- avoidance of prolonged use of hormones; and
- avoidance of excessive radiation exposure.

Sadly, even if it were possible to manage all of the risk factors that might theoretically be modified in some way, this would only lower the chance of having breast cancer by a maximum of 30%.

The fact that a person is a woman is the most significant risk factor for breast cancer. Men account for between 0.5 and 1 percent of all breast cancer cases. The management concepts used in the treatment of breast cancer in males are the same as those used in the treatment of breast cancer in women.

There is a correlation between having a family history of breast cancer and an increased chance of developing breast cancer oneself; nevertheless, the majority of women who are diagnosed with breast cancer have no family history of the illness. Even if there is no documented history of breast cancer in a woman's family, this does not always suggest that she is at a lower risk.

The majority of breast cancers are caused by mutations in the genes BRCA1, BRCA2, and PALB-2. Some hereditary gene mutations with "high penetrance" considerably enhance the chance of developing breast cancer. Women who have mutations in these important genes should carefully evaluate their options for lowering their cancer risk, which may include having both breasts surgically removed. The consideration of a strategy that is as highly intrusive as this one only applies to a very small number of women, and as such, it has to be thoroughly considered taking into consideration all of the available options.

TREATMENT

Treatment for breast cancer may be rather successful, with survival odds of 90% or higher when the illness is detected in its early stages. This is especially true when the cancer is treated. In most cases, treatment will involve some combination of surgery, radiation therapy, and anti-cancer drugs administered orally or intravenously in order to treat and/or lessen the likelihood of the cancer spreading to other parts of the body. This is referred to as locoregional control of the disease (metastasis). Endocrine treatment, often known as hormone therapy, chemotherapy, and, in rare instances, targeted biological therapy are all types of anti-cancer medications (antibodies).

In the past, surgical removal of the breast, known as a mastectomy, was the only option for treating breast cancer (complete removal of the breast). In cases when the cancer has spread extensively, a mastectomy may still be necessary. The majority of breast cancers may now be treated with a more limited operation known as a "lumpectomy" or partial mastectomy. In this technique, just the tumor is removed from the breast, and the rest of the breast is left intact. Radiation treatment to the breast is often necessary in these circumstances in order to reduce the risk of the cancer coming back in the breast.

During cancer surgery for invasive malignancies, lymph nodes are often removed as part of the procedure. In the past, it was believed that the only way to stop the progression of cancer was to do a full axillary dissection, which included removing all of the lymph node bed from beneath the arm. The term "sentinel node biopsy" refers to a less invasive lymph node operation that is now favoured since it has fewer potential consequences. This technique involves the use of dye and/or a radioactive tracer in order to locate the first few lymph nodes that the breast cancer might have progressed to.

The biological subtyping of breast cancers is used to determine the most appropriate medical therapies for the malignancies, which may be administered either before ("neoadjuvant") or after ("adjuvant") surgery. Endocrine (hormone) therapy, such as tamoxifen or aromatase inhibitors, are likely to be effective against cancers that express the estrogen receptor (ER) and/or progesterone receptor (PR). These drugs may be taken orally for anywhere between five and ten years, and they have been shown to cut the risk of recurrence of "hormone-positive" malignancies by almost half. Endocrine medications have the potential to bring on menopausal symptoms, although for the most part they are well tolerated.

The term "hormone receptor negative" refers to cancers that do not express ER or PR. These cancers must be treated with chemotherapy unless the malignancy is extremely tiny. The chemotherapy regimens that are available today are quite successful in lowering the likelihood of cancer spreading or returning, and outpatient chemotherapy treatment is often the most common delivery method. In the absence of difficulties, chemotherapy treatment for breast cancer often does not call for the patient to be admitted to the hospital.

A cancerous molecule known as the HER-2/neu oncogene may be overexpressed in breast tumors for unknown reasons. Cancers that test positive for the protein HER-2 may be treated with targeted biological medicines like trastuzumab.

Since they are antibodies rather than chemicals, these biological agents are exceedingly effective; nevertheless, this also means that they are quite costly. When targeted biological treatments are administered, they are often coupled with chemotherapy in order to boost each treatment's capacity to kill cancer cells.

The use of radiotherapy is also an extremely significant component of breast cancer treatment. Radiation therapy has the potential to save women diagnosed with breast cancer in its earlier stages the ordeal of having their breasts removed surgically. Even after a mastectomy has been done, patients with later-stage malignancies may benefit from radiation to lower their chance of a cancer recurrence. Radiation treatment has the potential to lessen the severity of breast cancer's later stages and, in certain cases, the risk of the patient passing away as a result of the illness.

THE IMPACT OF BREAST CANCER ON SURVIVORS?

1 . Emotional Impact: As a survivor of breast cancer, you may experience emotional changes such as depression and anxiety. You may also struggle with feeling guilty for surviving while others didn't or having difficulty trusting your body again. Coping with the emotional fallout of this disease is an important step in finding peace after breast cancer treatment and moving forward with life.

2. Physical Impact: The physical effects of breast cancer can be far-reaching, both during and after treatment. Some survivors find that they have less energy due to fatigue related to chemotherapy, radiation or other medical treatments. Others may experience pain, numbness or swelling in the

area where the tumor was removed leading to mobility issues or discomfort during everyday activities. Many women also experience menopause earlier than expected due to the hormonal changes brought about by breast cancer treatment.

3. Social Impact: Due to the physical and emotional changes that come with surviving breast cancer, many survivors also face social challenges such as being isolated from family and friends, feeling judged or misunderstood by those around them, or dealing with a sense of loss of autonomy due to their medical condition.

4. Financial Impact: Cancer treatment can be incredibly expensive, and many breast cancer survivors face the reality of financial strain due to medical bills and loss of income due to time off work to focus on their health.

5. Mental Health Impact: The mental health impact of breast cancer can be profound and

long-lasting. Many survivors find that they struggle with PTSD, panic attacks, or depression due to the traumatic experience of fighting and surviving a life-threatening illness such as this one. It's important to seek professional help if you are struggling emotionally and mentally in order to work through any issues that may arise.

6. Finding Balance: While the potential challenges faced by breast cancer survivors can be daunting, there is hope for finding balance and peace after such a long fight with this terrible disease. With proper care and support from medical professionals as well as loved ones, it is possible to move beyond breast cancer and find physical, mental, emotional, social and financial healing.

PART TWO:

LIVING BEYOND BREAST CANCER

PRACTICAL STEPS FOR RECOVERY AND LONG-TERM MANAGEMENT

As a breast cancer survivor, it can be difficult to know where to start when it comes to reclaiming your life after such an intense battle. Below are some practical steps that may help you along the path of recovery and long-term management:

1. Make time for self-care: Self-care is essential for post-cancer recovery and involves taking care of both physical and emotional health. This includes getting regular exercise, scheduling medical checkups, eating healthy foods, finding

ways to relax and manage stress levels, as well as making sure you're getting enough sleep each night. Additionally, consider joining support groups or attending counseling sessions with a mental health professional.

2. Embrace social support: Reaching out to family and friends can be an incredibly helpful way of coping with the trauma associated with cancer. Having a strong support system can be a major source of comfort, as well as provide support when making important decisions about your future health care.

3. Develop new interests: Finding activities that are enjoyable and meaningful is key in helping you adjust to life after breast cancer. Hobbies and activities such as yoga, gardening, painting, or playing music can help bring peace while providing an outlet for expressing emotions – both positive and negative. Additionally, pursuing

educational goals or engaging in volunteer work may offer renewed purpose in life.

4. Manage Cancer-Related Health Risks: This includes following recommended screenings for the recurrence of breast cancer, as well as managing other health conditions that may be linked to the disease. It's also important to take preventative measures by avoiding environmental toxins, eating a healthy diet, getting regular exercise, and reducing stress.

Following these steps can help you make it through the difficult journey of post-cancer recovery and ultimately find balance in life after breast cancer. With proper care and support from loved ones along with medical professionals who understand the unique needs of each survivor, living beyond breast cancer is possible – allowing us all to continue living our lives to the fullest.

EMOTIONAL SUPPORT FOR HEALING AND WELL BEING

1. Get Active

Regular exercise, such as yoga, can help reduce stress and anxiety and give you a sense of control over your body. You don't have to do a lot of exercises to achieve the benefits. Even simple activities, such as walking several times a week or practicing yoga, can lower stress and improve your quality of life.

2. Prioritize Self-Care

Focus on finding daily activities that not only make you feel good but also relieve stress and improve your well-being. Spending 10 minutes of quality time for you each day could mean reading a magazine, meditating, or playing with your pet.

Finding quiet moments in your day to reflect and quiet your mind, such as spending a few minutes in the car after you get home from work or running errands, can help you transition from the hectic pace of your day to being at home.

Meditating can be another helpful tool to prioritize time to relax and unwind. Mindfulness meditation uses specific breathing methods and may include guided imagery, as well as other relaxation and stress reduction techniques. Research shows mindfulness meditation may reduce stress, anxiety, and fear.

Other ways to lower stress and anxiety include journaling and listening to music.

3. Talk to Someone

Social support offers emotional support, practical help, and advice through interactions with people in your life, such as family members, friends, spiritual advisors, co-workers and supervisors, and healthcare providers.

You may feel more comfortable talking one-on-one with a counselor or therapist or prefer to only share your feelings and thoughts with close family and friends. Everyone has different needs. It's important to find a healthy support system that works for you.

For those who are comfortable, talking with a trained mental health provider, such as a psychiatrist, psychologist, counselor, or clinical social worker, can reduce stress and improve mental well-being and quality of life. Mental health counseling can combine techniques such as coping skills and relaxation exercises to help reduce stress.

4. Join a Support Group

Some people prefer one-on-one counseling, while others prefer counseling in a group setting.

Support groups can increase your network of people who can support you in your emotional health journey.

You may need to attend a support group a few times before you feel comfortable sharing with others or asking questions. Finding the right support group is essential. Be open-minded. You may need to try a few different support groups before finding the right one for you.

FINDING BALANCE IN LIFE AFTER TREATMENT

1 . Connect with the Right People: Finding friends, family, and healthcare professionals who understand the unique challenges faced by breast cancer survivors can be an invaluable source of support during this time. Having people to talk to or confide in can provide emotional relief, help discuss difficult topics, and offer a different perspective on life after cancer.

2. Exercise: Exercise is essential for overall health and well-being following treatment for breast cancer. Moderate physical activity can reduce fatigue, stress, and depression and improve quality of life while strengthening muscles and bones that may have been weakened by chemotherapy or radiation treatments.

3. Eat Well: Eating a nutritious diet rich in protein, fruits, and vegetables can help boost the immune system while promoting the healing of tissues damaged by treatment. Focusing on eating healthy foods, staying hydrated, and avoiding processed and high-sugar items can help reduce inflammation and provide energy.

4. Get Enough Rest: After cancer treatment, it is vital to make sure the body is getting enough sleep in order to rest and regenerate itself. Lack of proper rest can lead to fatigue, lack of focus, depression, and a weakened immune system so

making sure to get enough restful sleep should be a priority for all breast cancer survivors.

5. Find Joy in Life: Despite the challenges faced during treatment and beyond, there are still moments of joy that can be found during life after breast cancer. Whether it's spending time with loved ones or engaging in hobbies you enjoy – don't forget to take time to enjoy and appreciate life after cancer!

RECLAIMING JOY AND FULFILLMENT THROUGH NEW VENTURES

Life after breast cancer can be a time of trepidation and fear—but it can also be an opportunity to discover new passions and directions in life. Many survivors take this chance to develop hobbies or skills that they had always wanted to learn, such as cooking, painting, playing an instrument, or gardening. This can help them explore their creative side while also providing an outlet for stress relief. Whether big or small, these ventures into the unknown territory are essential steps on the road to recovery and finding peace in the aftermath of treatment.

Others take the chance to travel, explore new cultures and places, or take on volunteer activities that give back to their community. Becoming involved in a cause bigger than themselves can be empowering for breast cancer survivors—allowing them to tap into their courage and strength while finding joy and hope in life after cancer.

With proper support systems, understanding medical professionals, and loving family members and friends by their sides, many breast cancer survivors are able to find fulfillment through these new journeys. And with each step they take on this path towards recovery, they are reminded of the positive impact they have made not only on their own lives but also on those around them!

reclaiming joy and fulfillment in life after breast cancer. No matter the path a survivor takes, it is possible to find joy and peace of mind by embracing all that life has to offer. With proper care and support from medical professionals and loved ones, living beyond breast cancer can be a reality!

CONCLUSION

Life after breast cancer is attainable, and there are many ways to make this journey manageable. With the right support from those around them, survivors can find strength in their resilience to move forward. Physically and emotionally, it's important that cancer survivors take care of themselves and prioritize their own needs. This could mean seeking professional help or finding new activities that bring joy and peace of mind. It is possible to live beyond either a current diagnosis or after treatment, providing hope for anyone facing a similar battle in their life.

No matter what path you're on, remember that healing doesn't occur overnight – but every moment of strength is worth celebrating. Cancer survivors deserve respect, recognition, and love as they continue along their journey. With the right care and support, life after breast cancer can be full of hope and joy.

www.ingramcontent.com/pod-product-compliance
Lightning Source LLC
Chambersburg PA
CBHW071123220526
45467CB00004B/2027